FORTY POEMS*
FOR FORTY POUNDS
(*TO BE READ BY THE REFRIGERATOR LIGHT)

Publisher: Paul McGahren
Editorial Director: Kerri Grzybicki
Layout & Design: Jodie Delohery

Cedar Lane Press
PO Box 5424
Lancaster, PA 17606-5424

Paperback ISBN: 978-1-950934-67-6
ePub ISBN: 978-1-950934-70-6
Hardcover ISBN: 978-1-950934-81-2

Library of Congress Control Number: 2021933608

Printed in the United States of America
10 9 8 7 6 5 4 3 2 1

To learn more about Cedar Lane Press books, or to find a retailer near you, email Info@CedarLanePress.com or visit us at www.CedarLanePress.com.

FORTY POEMS*
FOR FORTY POUNDS
(*TO BE READ BY THE REFRIGERATOR LIGHT)

By Trish Dougherty

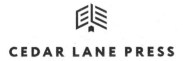

CEDAR LANE PRESS

For My Mother

FORTY POEMS

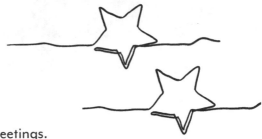

LIFETIME

Sometimes I miss the meetings.

I still have my gold star stickers
they were sweeter than cookies
more refreshing than beer—
I loved those stickers.

I buy sheets of them at the store
they aren't the same
they don't taste as sweet
not without a whole room of polite clapping
   to back them up

Now, I am alone,
just me and this lifetime of diet lore
just me and my daily log book
just me and my daily log book and early morning
   encounters with the bathroom scale
just me, the log book, the bathroom scale and these poems.

You're my gold star now, dear reader,
Share this with me.

(Polite clapping)

YOU ARE NOT ALONE

You are not alone as you stand before your mirror
sucking it in
pulling back your shoulders
posing.

You are not alone as you approach the scale
pulling off your socks
and jewelry
bracing.

You are not alone in your worries
cholesterol
high blood pressure
immobility.

I am right behind you
not weighing what my driver's license says
winded after climbing the stairs
depressed.

But it helps to know we are together
and there are so many of us.
Maybe instead of asking about a new friend's religion
or what kind of car they drive
we should just casually inquire,
"Do you weigh yourself nude?"

And when they say yes, we can throw our arms
    around them
and cry, and say sister
and laugh at our licenses together
and know that we are not alone.

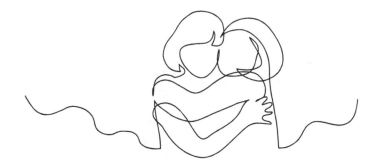

DIVINE INTERVENTION

I ruthlessly pruned a third of my wisteria
the magazines said that would make it bloom—
magazines are rubbish.

The measured snipping made me yearn
for the Master Gardener—
who would take His hand to me
coax out my flowers
and maybe do a little something about this
    unsightly spreading...

It's still early spring
too soon to tell
if I did any good for my wisteria
or accidentally killed the whole thing.

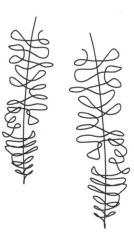

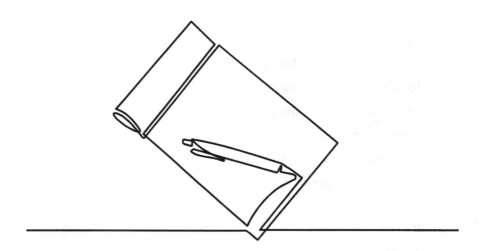

TOO MANY CONFESSIONS
ARE NOT GOOD EITHER

The act of starting a diet contains within it the confession
    that you are overweight.
"Sorry, I'm dieting," you whisper with a hand out to stop
    the food being pushed on you
and you whisper it
but the room echoes as if you shouted.

Diligently writing down every single thing you eat contains
    the confession that you don't pay attention.
Sometimes I write things down before I even eat them
just to see how they will play out.
It doesn't stop me
but it feels proactive.

Weighing your food is the confession that you lie.
What matters one gram when we are all going to
    die eventually?
It doesn't matter at all
write down what the kitchen scale says.

Weighing yourself is the confession that you can't see
    yourself.
I step on the platform but the number it shows is just one
    arbitrary axis.
I am immeasurable.

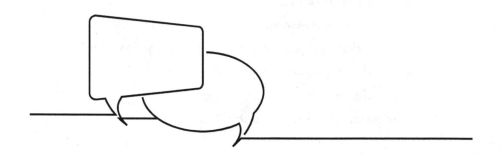

WHAT'S BEING SAID

I made this for you
so you have to eat it

You opened a package,
you shouldn't have, really.

I made   for you
so you have

Constantly with the "I."
followed by guilt,
Guilt and a threat.

I   for you
so you

You always think of food
     when you're worried,
as my body changes our
     relationship changes.

I   for
   you

You know my likes and dislikes,
     we have shared hundreds
     of meals
what will we share now?

I
   you

I'm not leaving you,
but it's your turn to be the
     fat friend.

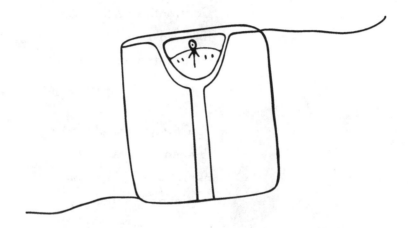

PLATEAUED

The scale will not change.
I nudge it to another part of the floor
where the slope is more treacherous.
I flip it one-hundred-eighty degrees
maybe the slope is benevolent now?
The scale will not change.

I'm trying to find a place in this tiny bathroom
where two plus two equals three.

In the future will houses come with special nooks
where gravity is weak?
A kitchen with a dark corner where all laws of biology and
    conservation of matter are helpfully suspended?

What future, I wonder,
as the scale does not change.

I CHEATED

I ate when I wasn't hungry

I ate because I was sad
I ate because I was a hole that needed to be filled
I ate because my mouth was empty

I ate my loneliness
I ate my streak of being good
I ate my self-respect

I ate garbage
I invented new freestyle garbage to eat
ham wrapped around bread wrapped around cheese
ham wrapped around fingers wrapped around thighs

I became garbage
sadder, lonelier and emptier
arms wrapped around shoulders wrapped around knees
grief wrapped around loneliness wrapped around nothing

REASONS

cheekbones as sharp as my tongue
that crease between my chins which never tans
the flaps on my arms that remind me
(and everyone else who sees them) of Grandma
seeing my feet without leaning
chub rub
tall boots
belts

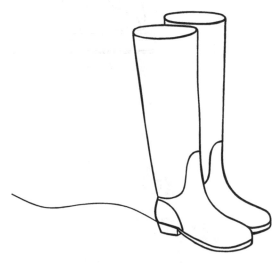

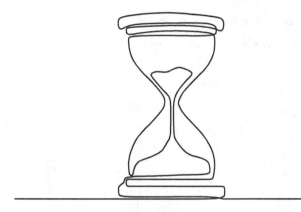

I'M OUT

It's two o'clock in the afternoon
and I am out of calories for the day—
out of sugar, out of sodium, out of fat.

My recommended daily allowance suggests
I now go sit in the corner
and think about my choices.

The next ten hours stretch out before me
like an ocean of weak herbal tea
studded with lemon wedges.

I will accept this,
(not quite as greedily as I accepted that cheeseburger
    and fries)
but stoically
and with head held high
I accept the consequences.

I knew what I was doing.
I knew it would be my last meal of the day.
I savored every bite
treasured every swallow—

it was better than ten thousand celery sticks.

THE MONSTER WITHIN

Even after I have dutifully voraciously consumed
    my breakfast
I can feel it
the gnawing and growling of my little monster.
This is what I make it, I decide.

"Eat me," I croon nudging a roll of flesh helpfully closer.
Should I name the monster, or would that be weird?

I already find myself looking for him
the same way I search out dumpster raccoon

And isn't this monster just the same?
Picking through my garbage
studying a thigh, decomposing it into all the bad choices
that contributed to that particular jiggle
judging the soft yeastiness, testing it with a nibble.

"Eat me," I whisper and offer myself up to the monster.
This isn't weird.

I wish he would take giant bites
the teasing, the imperceptible changes
frustrate me.

I want more violence
I want him to tear at this body
to pull away all that is soft and unnecessary
until I am hard.
Until I am a warrior.

That's what monsters are for—
the gnawing and growling intensify.
Good.

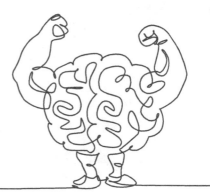

THIS YOU MUST DO

Strap sticks of butter to your thighs
feel them sliding and greasy—
take them off again and revisit how you lost that pound.

Tuck a bag of flour under your shirt
artisan flour in a generous cotton sack—
the flour loose and soft and white
then take it off and lose five pounds again.

The entire world has been weighed, measured, calibrated;
props are readily available.

A forty-pound bag of dog kibble
slides in my arms and the weight shifts suddenly
I heft the bag higher and dream of the day
of the fortieth poem.

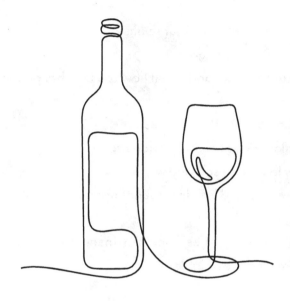

DECISIONS

I went to the grocery store after a long day of work
the list included such vagaries as
yogurt, cereal, ice cream and spaghetti sauce

by the time I reached the spaghetti sauce I was on
   the phone,
not in tears
but tear-adjacent.

Greek, low-fat, coconut—already negotiated;
four cereals: one chocolate, one novelty, one with
   strawberries, and raisin bran were in the cart;
two ice creams: espresso chip and chocolate peanut butter
   cup were slowly softening.

I stood there before a wall of red sauces
with no decisions left
a bankrupt puddle of crushed tomatoes.

I borrowed the strength of the voice on the phone
selecting a home-style marinara with onions and garlic
in a jar that held a pleasing shape
and turned my battered spirit toward the long, quiet,
   checkout lines.

But just then the voice continued, soft and full of love,
maybe you can get some wine too?

PRETENDING

thin young women
thin young women on TV
thin young women on TV dancing in tiny dresses
thin young women on TV dancing in tiny dresses
  and drinking with abandon

the thin young women on TV dancing in tiny dresses
  and drinking with abandon are pretend

don't try to be them, it will end in tears

pretend you are still young
pretend you are thin—
   you are thinner than you think
pretend your dress is a trendy slip of a thing, just like you.
pretend you have abandoned all your cares

but don't actually
life is not pretend;
it will end in tears

you don't need the drama
you don't need the huffing and fighting and gossiping
you don't need the empty calories of fifteen-dollar cocktails

maybe you do need the dancing
no matter what, it will end in tears

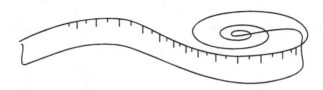

WHAT'S IN A SIZE?

I strut out of the dressing room triumphant,
which doesn't happen very often
not to me—not to anyone.

I am a 10, short and curvy.
The jeans I toss in the trash are not—
but now I am, check my size.

The strutting continues undiminished
through the grocery store
the checkout line.

The cashier asks to see my ID
she holds it close to study.

Do I really look that good...
or did I pick the cheapest wine?

The cashier types on her screen
updating my file no doubt
adding the new size.

The receipt includes my horoscope and a number to call
the coupons are for fancy shampoo
and a wine-tasting seminar.

The strutting continues, with blessings.

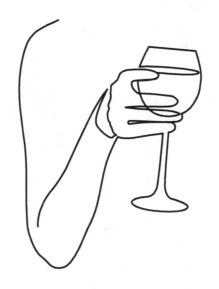

CHEAT DAY

The most sacred cheat day
and its holy restorative powers, amen,
pours a glass of red wine
at noon on the nose.

Plans a dinner with bread, with pasta,
with pork stuffed with pork.

This ever-glorious cheat day
includes a lot of trouble
a good deal of fussing
and some expense.

It's an event to work for
not something you're due
not an entitlement—
but an achievement.

The most sacred cheat day
and its holy restorative powers, amen,
pours a glass of red wine
and raises a toast to life—

remember this happiness
remember this joy
remember this feeling tomorrow.

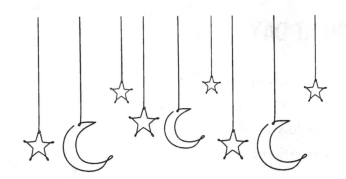

BEYOND NUMBER

Wheeling across the night sky the stars are
without number in their depth and glory

much like the crackers that I ate tonight.
Beyond count as I slipped them, one by one,
though some had cheese, into my waiting mouth.

Barely empty it was, as cracker followed cracker.
The beer could scarcely keep up
with the washing down the throat
with the swishing of the palate.

The stars bring their complexity and glory
wheeling across the night sky—
so grand, so aloof, so removed
from the thousand tiny hurts
and these thousand crackers.

Each a band-aid
each a bruise
each a mistake
without number
beyond counting
though some had cheese.

How can you ask me
to record the stars?

DAILY FIBER

Almost every product advertises them
the brothers fiber: soluble and insoluble

or by not proclaiming,
thus, declares an absence.

Also useful.

But where does one shop for moral fiber?
Which aisle does it lurk within?

I'm asking for a friend.
The same friend who put that ice cream in my cart.

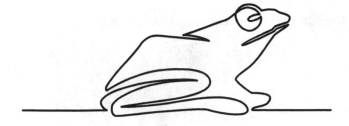

THE DEADLINE

An Event lurches into view on your horizon
a Most Auspicious Day that someone will need to capture.

The Group Photo is going to be blown up, up, up,
and hang on someone's wall,
  no matter
    how bad
      you look.

They will place you in the front row,
in the center of the front row shorty,
and fan out around you
like Flowers surrounding A Toad.

A date appears on the calendar
and suddenly everything is in focus
there is a clarity and an urgency that was missing before;

back when I was expecting that I could
  lose
    and regain
      the same two pounds
        forever.

It behooves us, my friends,
take advantage of this situation.

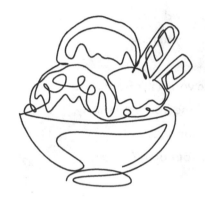

PULLING

In pottery class as I struggle to center my clay
(centering is hard)
Stacey asks what I'm making.
A tall slender vessel, I snarl, smacking and bullying the clay.

Later we will discuss which is the lowest form of pottery:
is it the humble salsa bowl or the cat food dish?

I watch another bowl spin on my wheel
refusing to be tall or slender
maybe I can fill this one with ice cream.

LOVE

Bread that you kneaded and nurtured and made
   from scratch,
that you pulled hot out of the oven
cut too soon, and slathered in butter
that's not love.

Chocolate chip cookies that require a trip for milk
barely cooked in the middle
spread hot and gooey
they are not love.

Homemade chicken soup, lasagnas and pot pies—
delicious and nurturing and lovely to share,
yes, yes, yes—
but not love.

You can love making them,
love the people you make them for
you can even make them with love

but they're food: amalgamations of fats and sugars.
An entirely different kind of chemistry
don't conflate the two.

Love is holding hands in the parking lot
Love is cuddling closer after you hit the snooze button
Love is gluten-free.

But I don't want to hurt your feelings, so I'll eat this
    anyway—
pass the milk.

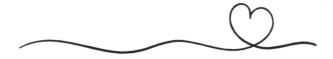

DIFFERENT

I look at my thighs spreading across the chair
like waves running up the shoreline
they spread and spread
filling all available space
covering as far as they can reach,
as far as the denim tide allows.

And I feel exactly the same.

I wish for all the pictures I deleted
so I can compare my neck
compare my cheeks
the depth of my eye sockets
has anything changed?

I feel exactly the same.

I fold jeans that are size eight instead of fourteen,
the fabric is the same blue.

I don't know what to feel.

Maybe someday I will feel confident
accomplished in this tiny thing that so many
    people manage.

Maybe someday my thighs will be acceptable
but I don't know how to get there
I don't know if this is the road that gets me there
or if I need to change something besides
the numbers on the scale.

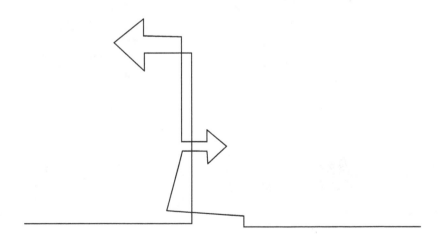

JUST ONE HAIKU

hole in my bagel
dripping with melted cream cheese
deduct calories.

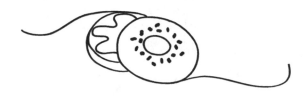

A FUNERAL AS SEEN FROM THE ACQUAINTANCE SECTION

Stand about midway back in the church—
not as far forward as family
not suspiciously in the back like some dramatic secret.

This is an old person's funeral
the tide of her life, which once surged forth,
ebbs away completely today.

Once upon a time she flew to California,
visited family, stuck her toe in the Pacific.
She used to slurp down clams on the beach
and all August long she smelled like tomatoes.

At the end her world was the kitchen chair,
the recliner
the bed.

She knew everyone at the co-op
was on the library board for years
dwindled to nurses and hospice volunteers.
Life went on without her
not noticing she was still around.

Kneel about halfway back in the church;
think about who might come to your funeral.
it's an odd expenditure of energy, thinking about
    your own funeral.

It's nice to have a few plans, spare others the burden
    of guessing...
you'll never know what happens.

A hundred people could show up
moved by the beauty of the obituary you prepared in advance.
Or maybe at the last minute, or now in a fit of whimsy,
you leave everything to your neighbor's niece.
The one who checks in on you,
brings you the good bread from the co-op
because she remembers seeing you there squeezing the loaves
    looking for crust.

One day she asked, and you tore off the end,
right there in the store, just ripped it off and handed it over
so she could taste
(it was a very good loaf with a crust that crackled
and a crumb you could chew).

You leave it all to her with instructions:
no funeral, no empty church pews,
no flowers thrown on a grave like sacrificial Greek lovers,
sell what you can
give away what you want.

Visit Italy
eat the good bread for me
life is in the memory of food we share.

You're standing now, flipping hastily through the hymnal
already a verse behind
it's hard to read with the tears streaming down.

BON APPÉTIT

slick pages hold all of my attention
I linger over two-page spreads

studying the captions, the details,
every morsel of information

I have to swallow before turning the page
swallow and take a deep breath

the next image is the most captivating yet
in such detail that I can smell it

I'm hot and dizzy
not sure I can bear to turn the page again

cookbooks have replaced romance novels
food magazines are the new pornography

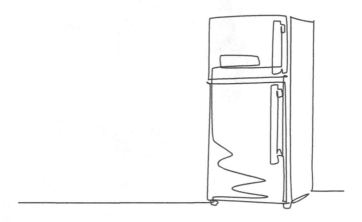

SECRETS

Standing in the shame-filled glow of the refrigerator.

Casing the options before me:
repurposed margarine tub, Tupperware, pie plate.

Who turns their nose up at cold sweet potatoes
served fresh (or maybe not so fresh)
from the fridge at ten o'clock at night?

Are they refusing the cranberry sauce too?
And this perfectly good quarter slice of pie?

Close all the lids and return them to their shelves.
Wash and dry the spoon, tuck it back in the drawer.
It was too few bites to bother writing down.

This never happened.

SNOBS

There are enough people who don't appreciate
the nice things, we don't need to cultivate them.

Husband says I have done a disservice to my sons
offering them the most delicious food.

I think it more tragic to accept bland sustenance,
dutifully consuming rote calories for the sake of survival.

Should I have taught them to live with bare walls?
Provided cells without books or soft chairs?

Should I have raised Spartans without gardens
who can't tell a daffodil from a rose?

My children know a Monet from a Seurat
and a Mornay from a Hollandaise

they were raised in my petite salon
to be ideal dinner companions.

They expect pillows, and blankets,
home-baked cookies served warm with milk.

If that makes them snobs, unsuited for life
in this harsh bleak world, they can always stay with me.

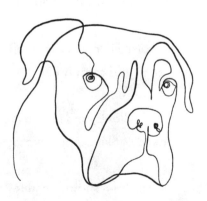

AN ASSIST

The clattering of a spoon breaks me
out of my early morning lethargy,
that son-of-a-bitch dog is eating my breakfast.

I could measure out a new bowl,
it doesn't matter much—
   none of this matters—
but the bathroom scale was unkind—
   let us not speak of it.

Perhaps this is the universe
bending low, lending a hand or a paw,
or really, an opportunistic licking.

So I content myself
with moping about the trials of dieting
and poorly trained Boxers.

Lamenting the things that are within your power
to change, to improve—
   really, everything is there you can pour another bowl—
it's unattractive.
Take the assist and move on with your morning.

CHERRY CHIP

This is the bowl of ice cream
that I ate when you said you weren't coming back.
Cherry vanilla, soft and sweet like you used to be.

The brittle chocolate bits breaking under my teeth
were me.
The cherries, cold and frozen,
were your wretched little heart, doing this to me.

I swirled it with the smallest spoon
so that each bite could have both of us together again.

Then I stood there, slumped over the counter,
reading your email again and again
long after the ice cream was gone.

HURTING

I want to spread every feeling
across hot buttered toast
and eat and eat forever.

Grow as big as a house
the biggest ever
so everyone can see
how much I'm hurting.

And I want to never eat again.
Sew my lips shut
hold up a hand
and shake my head
no, no, no.

Never eat again
and look so thin, so tragic
that everyone can see
how much I'm hurting.

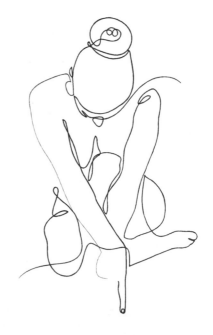

MAYBE

Maybe this is the definition of growing up:
realizing that if I had a magic wand
and waved it to be a size two it wouldn't last.

Quick fixes are temporary
sooner or later we slide back
to what we've always been,

the young come along and chide us
call us complacent and pessimistic—
the word they're looking for is pragmatic.

Maybe this is the point of growing up:
mapping the parameters of your comfort zone
and finding the sweet spot
corners you don't mind cutting
a reflection you don't mind seeing.

Maybe this is the wisdom of growing up:
seeing things beyond the surface
accepting my own shortcomings
so I can empathize with others.

Maybe I'm too old for this.

ANDY CAPP FRIES

Sitting in a bar with new friends
the spicy not-too-hot flavor from this bowl of French fries
transports me back to my first bar.

Murphy's didn't believe in food
only tiny bags of Andy Capp Fries.

It was a bar so unadorned
my mother refused to go in and fetch my father
she sent me instead.

I had to stop just inside the door,
wait for my eyes to adjust from the dazzling
    summer sunlight
to the dim space.

I remember standing there caught in the darkness
knowing the men could all see me.

I remember the tall black vinyl stools
perching with my grandfather and my father
trying not to stare at the man with no nose.

My father died first.
The bar closed second.
But my grandfather had already stopped going there.

We lost more than my father that year
we lost everything he loved too because it all hurt so much.

My grandfather died a long time later.
I have no idea when the man with no nose died.

The next time I order these fries
I will think of them all again, forever in their regular spots.
Forever smiling as they wait for my eyes to adjust,
as they wait for me to run to them.

And for that I am grateful—
food is a gift.

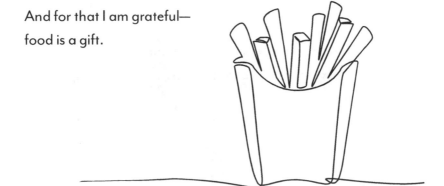

REMIND ME

When life gets dark remind me I have a cannoli in my purse.

Remind me about the joy that comes from chasing
    a two-year-old
snatching them up and holding them close, tickling
    and shrieking.

Remind me how your arm feels when it slides along
    the dip of my waist,
skin soft and bare touching skin soft and bare.

Help me remember the feeling of lake water closing
    over my head;
popping up again hair slicked back, eyes as dark as a seal.

Remember dancing, I'm terrible at dancing but sometimes,
when the music is loud enough, I forget and do it anyway.

Remember getting lost in the city, but making good time
   doing it.
Holding hands and marching downtown with the lights,
   block after block.

I don't want to eat it—I don't ever need to eat it—
But when life gets dark, remind me, I have a cannoli in
   my purse.

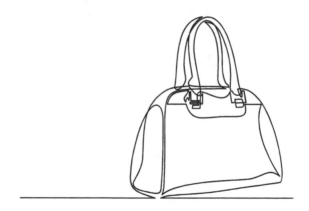

TROY, IF HELEN WAS A PIZZA

My food diary stretches back six months now
long enough to be a siege.

Like any good war I have no recollection of how it started,
was there a word spoken out of turn
or has this been the whim of a god?

In my battle I imagine the Greeks bear promises
    of health and happiness;
the Trojans hunker down with warm buttered toast
    and ignore them.
I am both sides.

I think about Patroklos trying to wear a better man's armor,
and dying in it on the field outside the gates.
I worry about being struck down by a spear
before I can eat ice cream again.

I am Odysseus, quick with savage planning and canny
    bartering
as I struggle to not give up, to gain whatever ground I can.
It's the Trojans that let strange food into my city.

I am Penelope too,
obediently industrious all day in front of the suitors
but alone, at night, everything is undone.
At night the loneliness creeps up my throat
and wine chases it back down.

This food diary tells a tale
as clear as Achilles' shield, though not quite as dark,
the empty plains of repeated meals are, cruelly,
    the triumphs
parties and friends mark lost ground.

(The irony lends itself to a balance
And the endurance of the siege.)

This rocky plateau I have named Scylla,
that vortex of emotional eating is Charybdis,
the way through is tricky and prone to backsliding.

I have a weight log too—
recorded in private
in the nude
in the bathroom.

The graph shows a wandering star,
drifting close to a goal then shooting away again
drawing near and drawing back.

I can reach a weight and hold it,
hold close to it for a few weeks as the numbers
    become familiar,
master that weight and then reach out for the next one.

It's slow,
so slow this way,
but maybe it's sustainable.

Back and forth the siege continues;
will it be ten years,
twenty years,
the rest of my life?

I am Calypso,
enraptured with the project,
holding myself captive.

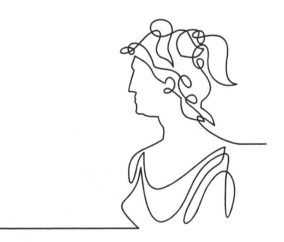

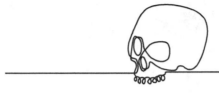

BONES

The scale looms before me and
I don't want to get on it.

I just want to sit here
alone on the bathroom floor
and put my head down
and cry for a hundred years

then you can come in
and weigh my dry white bones
and take my measure

then

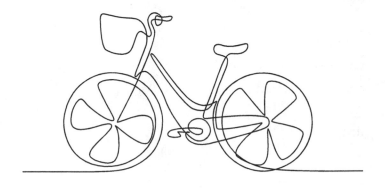

PRAISE

There are times where the mother
stands behind the bicycle cheering and clapping.

There are times where the mother
peeks through the door, steps away again.
Her praise isn't required for every single thing.

I don't know if I have ever tried to explain this to you.

There are times when what you're doing
has to be for your own reasons.
Parenting guides call them natural consequences;
parenting teachers ask if we want to raise autonomous
   adults
or not

There are times we do.

There are times, when I'm not sure
I want to be
an autonomous adult.

I spy you
spying on me.
Run behind my bicycle
stomping your feet
waving your hands in the air
shouting so everyone hears,
"Your ass looks fabulous Mom!"

SPRING

tender thin green hands
gently remove sweaters

the humid exhales of the earth
push up the hem of my pants

wrists and ankles are bared
forearms and calves, elbows and knees

like a receding tide
the warmth rushes over me

this is not the body
that I put to bed last fall

it's as new as the grass
as fresh as a flower

I greet it like the sun greets the morning
Hello knees!

I put sandals on and pose in front of the mirror
a t-shirt so old it's new again fits again
drawers are emptied
the pile on the bed grows and cascades to the floor

it's spring
and the world
fits me

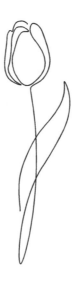

ENGINEERS

They say there are not enough women engineers
and yet every summer scores of us put on bathing suits.

The geometry of conic sections;
the rigging of straps artfully lifting;
tensile strength of space-age fabrics
cunningly woven with camouflaging puckers,
camouflaging panels and lines,
camouflaging everything.

All of that measured against price,
against color, against availability.

All of that considered against the challenges of the day:
the venue, the audience, the potential athletic demands.

All of that taken against the goal—
which is never to look good—
but realistically
to just look the best one can reasonably expect
and to be comfortable with that.

They say there are not enough women engineers...
maybe they don't know where to look.

MISTAKES

Twenty-five-cent hot dog night at the local ball park:
attending was a mistake,
bringing my own mustard was not.

I baked a lasagna when I was home alone;
completely unsupervised with fifteen pounds
of hot and bubbling deliciousness.

I planted mint straight in the ground
in my garden.
I'll just drink that many mojitos I bragged,
like a fool.

I saw the same movie three times
because the theater served beer and burritos
cried every time too.

I ordered a five-gallon tin of cheese popcorn,
my son dared me to.
Right after I dared him to dare me.

I was also the 'winning' high bid for a case of
    cheese popcorn,
it was for charity.
Charitable eating is still eating.

Cheese popcorn is my weakness
so is beer
and pizza
and life.

What can you do?

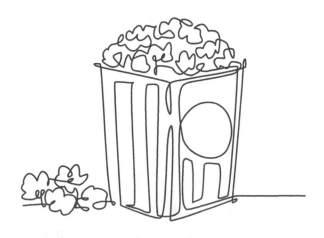

SKIN

As you rush through life
hands creaking on the steering wheel,
remember to breathe—
remember to enjoy the skin you're in

fill your skin,
be you as you are now

not an old shirt
stretched out
unflattering

not a future shirt
buttons gaping
too tight to move

wear the thing that fits you now
wear it every single day

no one minds

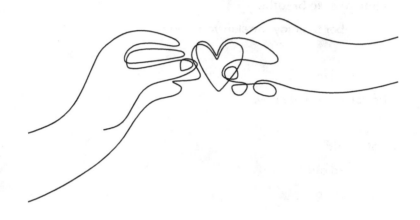

THERE IS NO FORTIETH POEM

There is no happy ending
no ending at all.

Only different degrees of caring
and paying attention, of diligence.

I wish you enough family photo events
to keep you from wandering too far.

I wish you long plateaus
close to where you want to be.

I wish you friends to love and support you,
and failing that—

I'm glad you found this book.

TITLE INDEX

ABOUT THE AUTHOR

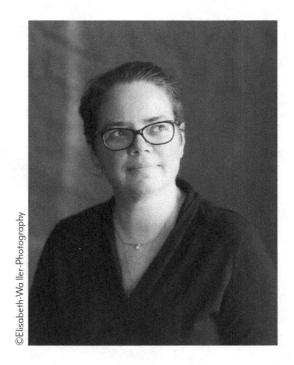

Trish Dougherty is a poet, mother & operator of the Beautiful Fairy Print Press. She is pursuing her post-graduate degree through Bread Loaf School of English.